BREAKING THE CHAINS OF SICKLE CELL DISEASES

DISEASES

(Advancements In the Treatment of Sickle Cell Disease)

BY

SHAWN B. KATE

Table of Contents

CHAPTER 1: INTRODUCTION

Sickle cell disease, a hereditary blood condition that affects millions of people worldwide, has been a silent foe for decades. This illness's history is one of suffering and persistence; it is a testament to human tenacity in the face of adversity. In this book, we set out on a journey to explore the remarkable advancements in the treatment of sickle cell disease, illuminating the steps taken to lessen the suffering of those affected.

Sickle cell disease has its roots in regions with an endemic malaria problem. Malaria is more common in some regions of the world, particularly in sub-Saharan Africa, because of a genetic mutation that imparts a degree of resistance to the disease. The trajectory of human history and genetics have been impacted by this complex genetic interplay, creating an interesting enigma that researchers have fought tirelessly to solve.

In the past, people with sickle cell disease had a very poor prognosis. The sickle- or crescent-shaped red blood cells that develop as a result of this sickness make them stiff and sticky. This alteration in shape causes the cells to become entangled in the blood vessels, which can cause organ damage, severe pain crises, and a host of other problems.

For many years, treating the symptoms and side effects of sickle cell disease was the main emphasis of treatment. The few options included hydroxyurea, pain medication, and blood transfusions. Although these treatments provided some relief, they did not address the underlying genetic defect that caused the illness. The incredible advancements made recently will be revealed when we delve deeper into this book. For people with sickle cell disease and their families, new pathways of hope have been made possible by advancements in genetics, biotechnology, and medical research. The range of available treatments is growing at an unheard-of rate, thanks to gene therapy and cutting-edge medications.

In the chapters that follow, we'll examine the sickle cell disease's historical setting, delve into the disease's intricacy, and trace the course of conventional treatments. The astounding advances in drugs, gene treatment, and emerging technology will be the subject of our next investigation. Along the way, we'll assess how these advancements have improved patients' quality of life and look at ongoing research projects that point to an even more promising future. The long-lasting darkness that sickle cell disease has put over the lives of those it affects is now starting to fade. Join us on this journey as we see the evolution of sickle cell disease therapy and the beginning of a brand-new age brimming with possibilities and optimism.

I sincerely hope you enjoy and learn a lot from this first chapter of your book. Please ask if you have any unique requirements or require additional help.

CHAPTER 2: HISTORICAL PERSPECTIVE

Genetics, medicine, and human perseverance are all woven into the tapestry of sickle cell disease history. We must first go back in time to understand the causes of this complex condition and the difficulties faced by those who dealt with it throughout history to fully understand the advancements in its treatment.

The Sickle Cell Disease's Discovery:

The early 20th century saw the first detection and description of sickle cell disease. When James B. Herrick, a dental student, examined the blood of a dental patient from the Caribbean in 1910, he noticed something important. Little did he know that this discovery would lead to the unraveling of a genetic blood ailment that would affect millions. He observed unusually shaped red blood cells under the microscope and described them as "sickle-shaped."

Genetics and Passivity:

Scientists started to comprehend the genetic causes of sickle cell disease as research progressed. It became clear that this condition was inherited autosomally recessively, which means that for a child to have the condition, both parents must possess a copy of the defective gene. This genetic finding made it possible to better understand why some individuals were more susceptible to the disease than others, particularly those who originated from regions where malaria was endemic.

Historical Difficulties:

People with sickle cell disease have faced several challenges throughout history. Medical care was at best rudimentary, and stigmatization and misunderstanding were pervasive. People impacted by pain crises, infections, and consequences typically lived shorter lives and had lower quality of life.

The Function of Malaria:

The history of sickle cell disease is notable for its connection to malaria prevention. It was discovered that persons with the sickle cell trait also known as the sickle cell gene had a higher chance of surviving in areas with a high malaria incidence. Further investigation into the underlying genetic causes of the uncommon association between malaria and sickle cell disease has resulted.

Inventive Scientists:

Pioneering researchers like Linus Pauling investigated the molecular causes of sickle cell disease as the 20th century went on. Pauling's research led to the conclusion that a mutation in the beta-globin gene was the disease's primary cause. This breakthrough paved the way for improved genetic knowledge and, eventually, tailored therapies.

The Path to Improvements:

The history of sickle cell disease is marked by a persistent search for information and treatments. In contrast to the early years, which were characterized by limited knowledge and therapeutic alternatives, significant advancements in pain control, supportive care, and the introduction of hydroxyurea as a therapy option were made in the second half of the 20th century.

We shall examine how these historical roots paved the path for the enormous advances in sickle cell disease therapy that we experience today in the chapters to come. The science, medicine, and personal experiences that have shaped the landscape of sickle cell disease treatment will be covered. As the pages of history are turned, we find ourselves on the cusp of a new era, one in which the

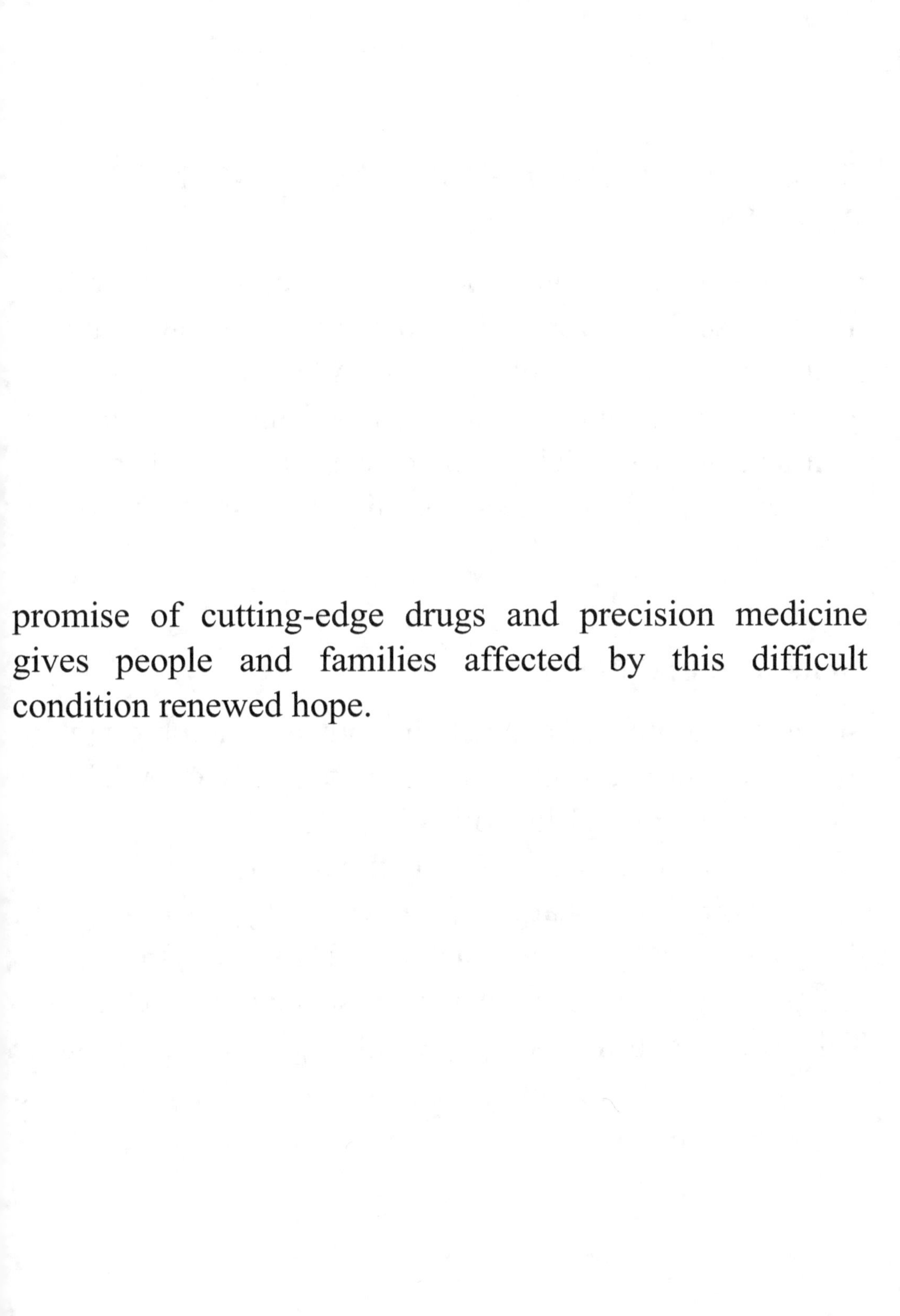

promise of cutting-edge drugs and precision medicine gives people and families affected by this difficult condition renewed hope.

CHAPTER 3: UNDERSTANDING SICKLE CELL DISEASE

It is essential to have a thorough understanding of the illness itself to appreciate the advancements in the treatment of sickle cell disease. We will examine the genetic basis, underlying mechanisms, and clinical manifestations of sickle cell disease in this chapter, as well as how they affect the lives of those who are affected.

Genetic Foundations:

Sickle cell disease is a genetic blood condition brought on by a specific beta-globin gene mutation. Hemoglobin S (HbS), an abnormal hemoglobin, is produced as a result of this mutation. The protein in red blood cells called hemoglobin is in charge of carrying oxygen throughout the body. In people with sickle cell disease, HbS makes red blood cells lose oxygen in a special "sickle" shape. This aberrant form makes the cells rigid and more prone to become tangled in blood vessels, which causes a variety of problems.

Recessive Autosomal Inheritance:

It is crucial to comprehend the genetics of sickle cell disease. It has an autosomal recessive inheritance pattern, which means that for a kid to be affected, they must receive two copies of the problematic gene from each parent. Sickle cell trait, which typically does not cause the disease but can be passed on to subsequent generations, is present in people who have one normal copy of the gene and one mutant copy.

Clinical Signs and Symptoms:

Numerous clinical symptoms of sickle cell disease might vary in intensity from person to person. Recurrent pain crises, which happen when sickled red blood cells clog blood vessels and cause excruciating agony, are the characteristic trait. Anemia, organ damage, and an increased risk of infections are further issues. Additionally, some people may experience acute chest syndrome, a stroke, or splenic injury.

Inheritance and Modifiers:

The variability of sickle cell disease is one striking feature. The genetic mutation that causes the illness is the same in all patients, although the intensity and frequency of the effects might vary substantially. Researchers have discovered genetic modifiers and additional factors that affect how the disease develops, shedding light on why some people experience milder symptoms while others struggle with more serious problems.

New Learnings from the Research:

Our knowledge of sickle cell disease has improved as a result of recent genetic and molecular biological discoveries. Scientists are uncovering the intricate molecular mechanisms involved in the development of disease, offering fresh targets for curative treatments. These discoveries raise the possibility of more precise treatment according to the unique genetic profiles of sickle cell disease sufferers.

Experiencing a Patient:

It's critical to address the human aspect of sickle cell disease in addition to the clinical aspects. Patients and their families frequently travel a difficult path of pain management, healthcare accessibility, and the psychological burden of dealing with a chronic illness. Their experiences offer a crucial context for understanding the struggles and victories associated with living with sickle cell disease. Through the course of this book, we'll examine how this deep understanding of sickle cell disease—from its genetic roots to its clinical manifestations—has opened the way for cutting-edge cures and therapies. The road taken to improve the lives of those affected by this affliction is a tribute to the power of medical advancement, scientific advancement, and the tenacious spirit of persons with sickle cell disease.

CHAPTER 4: STANDARD TREATMENT METHODS

Medical professionals and researchers have long depended on conventional therapy methods to decrease the burden of sickle cell disease. Despite not being curative, these methods have been crucial in reducing the condition's symptoms and side effects. The conventional methods and treatments that have served as the cornerstone of sickle cell disease management for many years will be covered in this chapter.

Pain Control:

Vaso-occlusive crises, commonly referred to as pain crises, are one of the most challenging aspects of sickle cell disease. These crises, which are characterized by excruciating agony, are brought on by sickled red blood cells blocking blood vessels. Pain management has been crucial to the treatment of sickle cell disease to address this. During times of crisis, pain is frequently treated with non-opioid and opioid medications, such as NSAIDs and opioids. However, the opioid problem has sparked further efforts to find alternative methods of pain treatment.

Hydrea (Hydroxyurea) and Hydration:

Dehydration can trigger or exacerbate crises in people with sickle cell disease, thus it's important to maintain adequate hydration. A medication called hydroxyurea, sometimes referred to as hydrea, has been used for many years to lessen the frequency and intensity of pain crises. It functions by promoting the development of fetal hemoglobin, which is less likely to sickle. Many people's lives have been significantly improved by hydrea as a treatment for sickle cell disease.

Transfusions of blood:

Another important part of the treatment for sickle cell disease has been blood transfusions. Red blood cell transfusions can increase the blood's ability to carry oxygen, lowering the risk of complications such as acute chest syndrome and stroke. However, repeated transfusions can cause iron overload, necessitating further treatments like chelation therapy to get rid of superfluous iron from the body.

Preventive measures and antibiotics:

Patients with sickle cell disease frequently get prophylactic antibiotics to avoid bacterial infections due to their increased susceptibility to infections, especially in children. To reduce the risk of developing a serious illness, vaccination against illnesses like pneumococcus and annual influenza vaccines are advised.

Supportive treatment and instruction:

Supportive care and patient education are essential components of a holistic approach to the management of sickle cell disease. This includes providing dietary support, emotional support, and instruction on symptom awareness and self-care. Improving overall health outcomes requires educating patients and their families.

While these conventional therapy approaches have been crucial in managing the illness, they do not address the genetic defect that results in abnormal hemoglobin synthesis, which is sickle cell disease's core cause. The subject of sickle cell disease treatment has seen a paradigm shift recently as researchers have concentrated on creating specialized medications and treatments meant to correct or alter genetic defects.

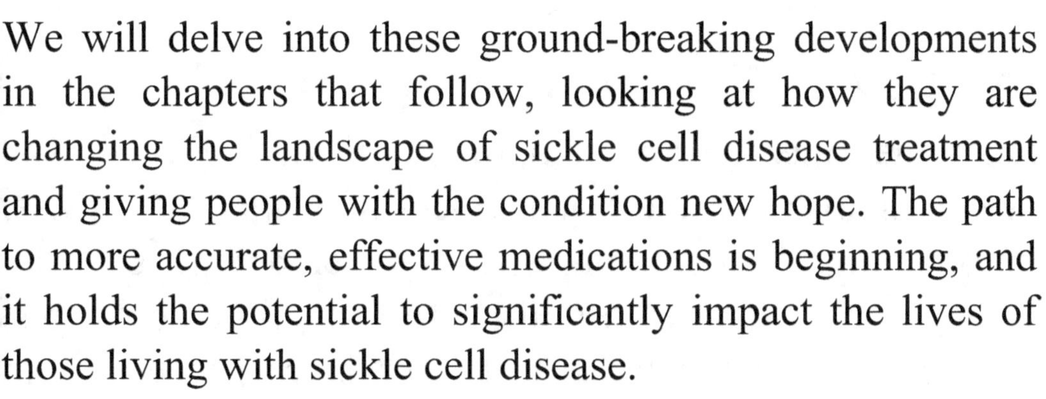

We will delve into these ground-breaking developments in the chapters that follow, looking at how they are changing the landscape of sickle cell disease treatment and giving people with the condition new hope. The path to more accurate, effective medications is beginning, and it holds the potential to significantly impact the lives of those living with sickle cell disease.

CHAPTER 5: ADVANCEMENTS IN MEDICINE

Recent advancements in medications specifically designed to address the disease's underlying causes have significantly changed the therapeutic landscape for sickle cell disease. In this chapter, we'll look into these ground-breaking pharmacological treatments that could significantly improve the quality of life for those with sickle cell disease.

Hydroxyurea (Hydrea):

For some time, hydroxyurea, often known as Hydrea, has been a mainstay in the management of sickle cell disease. It functions by promoting the development of fetal hemoglobin, which is less likely to sickle. By doing this, it lessens the frequency, severity, and other effects of pain crises. Hydroxyurea has changed the game by providing a reasonably simple and effective method to manage the condition.

L-glutamine Powder for Oral Use (Endari):

In 2017, the FDA authorized Endari, an oral powder form of L-glutamine, as a treatment for sickle cell disease. It functions by reducing oxidative stress, which aids in the development of sickled red blood cells. Clinical studies have shown that Endari can reduce the frequency of pain crises and improve patients' overall quality of life.

Oxbryta's Voxelotor:

Another drug that has been approved by the FDA for the treatment of sickle cell disease is voxelotor, which is marketed under the brand name Oxbryta. This medication increases hemoglobin's affinity for oxygen, preventing the development of sickled red blood cells. With the potential for improved oxygen delivery and fewer effects, Oxbryta represents a significant advancement in the treatment of the illness.

Clinical trials and fresh methods:

Clinical trials are being conducted on new agents and therapies in addition to the medications that the FDA has approved. These studies seek to address a variety of aspects of the illness, including reducing inflammation, enhancing blood flow, and lessening negative effects. The results of these trials could pave the door for brand-new therapeutic avenues and offer hope to people with sickle cell disease.

Precision therapies and personalized medicine:

Genetic advancements have also opened the possibility of personalized treatment options for sickle cell disease. Clinicians can modify treatment methods to increase effectiveness and minimize side effects by studying each patient's particular genetic profile. This method has a great deal of potential for improving care for each patient.

The pharmacological developments discussed in this chapter represent a significant change in the way sickle cell disease is treated. Even while there is still more to be done, the recent progress gives people and families affected by this difficult condition renewed hope and a brighter future. As we proceed through the other chapters, we'll learn about even more cutting-edge medical advancements and cutting-edge medicines with the potential to improve the quality of life for people with sickle cell disease.

CHAPTER 6: EMERGING TECHNOLOGIES AND GENE THERAPY

The world of medical research and innovation has embarked on a journey into the field of gene therapy and cutting-edge technology in quest of efficient treatments and perhaps potential cures for sickle cell disease. The innovative developments in gene therapy and emerging technologies that have the potential to improve the lives of people with sickle cell disease will be covered in this chapter.

Correcting the Genetic Mutation Through Gene Therapy:

By focusing on the genetic mutation that results in the production of faulty hemoglobin, gene therapy is a novel method of treating sickle cell disease. Numerous methods have been developed by researchers to correct or alter the genetic defect. One method is transferring corrected genetic material into a patient's bone marrow stem cells using viral vectors. This may result in the production of healthy, disease-free red blood cells.

Gene editing with CRISPR-Cas9:

With the development of CRISPR-Cas9 technology, the possibility of precise gene editing in sickle cell disease has increased. With the use of this new method, medical professionals can make precise changes to a patient's DNA, perhaps correcting the disease-causing gene. The use of CRISPR-based gene editing to treat sickle cell anemia is now being tested in clinical trials to determine its safety and effectiveness.

Gene-adding Treatment:

Transferring a functional copy of the healthy hemoglobin gene to a patient's cells is another method of gene therapy. By promoting the growth of healthy hemoglobin, this addition can lessen the prevalence of sickled red blood cells. Gene addition therapies are being studied and have shown promise in preliminary research.

News Monitoring and Diagnosis Technologies:

Beyond gene treatment, technological advancements are also altering how sickle cell disease is diagnosed and tracked. Blood tests, imaging, and wearable technology advancements are making it possible to diagnose issues and treat the illness more effectively. These innovations give patients better results and the chance for earlier intervention.

Transplantation of stem cells:

In certain instances, sickle cell disease has been cured with the use of stem cell transplantation, more especially allogeneic stem cell transplantation from a healthy donor. In this procedure, healthy donor bone marrow, which can produce normal red blood cells, is used to replace the patient's bone marrow. Although extremely effective, this treatment is challenging and risky, hence it is best suited for a small number of patients.

Issues and Proposed Courses of Action:

Although the developments in gene therapy and new technology are encouraging, challenges still exist. These include obstacles related to cost, accessibility, and safety. Researchers are continually working to get over these restrictions and improve these medications so they can be used more widely. To advance, researchers, medical experts, and patient advocacy organizations must work together constantly.

It becomes clear that a new era in the treatment of sickle cell disease is just around the corner as we delve deeper into the potential of gene therapy and cutting-edge technologies. Renewing optimism for those with this condition and their families is the promise of curative medications and more efficient disease management. The chapters that come after this one will continue to examine cutting-edge medical investigation and inventiveness in the fight against sickle cell disease.

CHAPTER 7: IMPROVING PATIENTS' QUALITY OF LIFE

Though advancements in therapies and treatments are important, improving the quality of life for people with sickle cell disease goes beyond medical solutions. In this chapter, we'll look at the various methods and approaches designed to improve patients' and their families' general health and quality of life.

Crisis Prevention and Pain Management:

The control of pain crises is one of the most important issues facing sickle cell disease patients. Enhancing quality of life requires not only managing pain but also avoiding crises through medication, hydration, and dietary changes. Multidisciplinary pain treatment teams collaborate closely with patients to develop procedures that are tailored to their individual needs.

Integrated Care:

Sickle cell illness frequently manifests with a range of effects on several organ systems. Treatment for these issues is provided by multidisciplinary care teams made up of hematologists, pulmonologists, cardiologists, and others. Regular check-ups and screenings aid in identifying problems early and produce better results.

Educating the Patient:

It is crucial to educate patients and their families about the disease. Education enables people to recognize symptoms, comprehend their illness, and make wise healthcare decisions. In providing resources and emotional support, patient advocacy groups and support networks can play a critical role.

Psychological Assistance:

A chronic condition like sickle cell disease can hurt a person's mental health. Patients frequently face emotional and psychological challenges in addition to physical ones. Counseling and assistance can be provided by mental health professionals to treat the disease's emotional components.

Care During Transition:

The healthcare system must adapt to the changing needs of adults with sickle cell disease as they enter adulthood. Young adults who are transitioning from pediatric to adult healthcare services can get aid from specialized transitional care programs.

Reducing Barriers to Care:

For the correct management of sickle cell disease, access to quality medical care is essential. Campaigning for laws that guarantee equitable access to medicines, therapies, and specialists is one way to improve access. Telemedicine, which enables remote access to medical treatments, has also become more and more important.

Trials in the Clinic and Research:

Individuals can expand their understanding of sickle cell disease and available treatment options by taking part in clinical trials and research studies. These studies offer a sense of purpose in the battle against the disease in addition to providing possible access to cutting-edge medicines.

Engagement in the Community and Advocacy:

To increase understanding, advance research, and advocate for the needs of people with sickle cell disease, patient advocacy groups and community involvement initiatives are essential. These initiatives raise the voices of those who are affected and bring about positive change.

Measures of quality of life:

Measurement and improvement of sickle cell disease patients' overall quality of life are increasingly the focus of research. Healthcare professionals can modify care plans using quality-of-life assessments to better meet the requirements of individual patients and improve their overall well-being.

Cultural Sensitivity:

To provide excellent care, it is essential to acknowledge and respect the cultural backgrounds and values of patients and their families. The provision of care is guaranteed to be sensitive and courteous thanks to cultural competency.

Remembering that improving patients' quality of life is at the core of our efforts to advance sickle cell disease treatment is vital. Beyond medical advancements, comprehensive care, support systems, and advocacy are what significantly improve the lives of people and families affected by this condition. In the chapters that

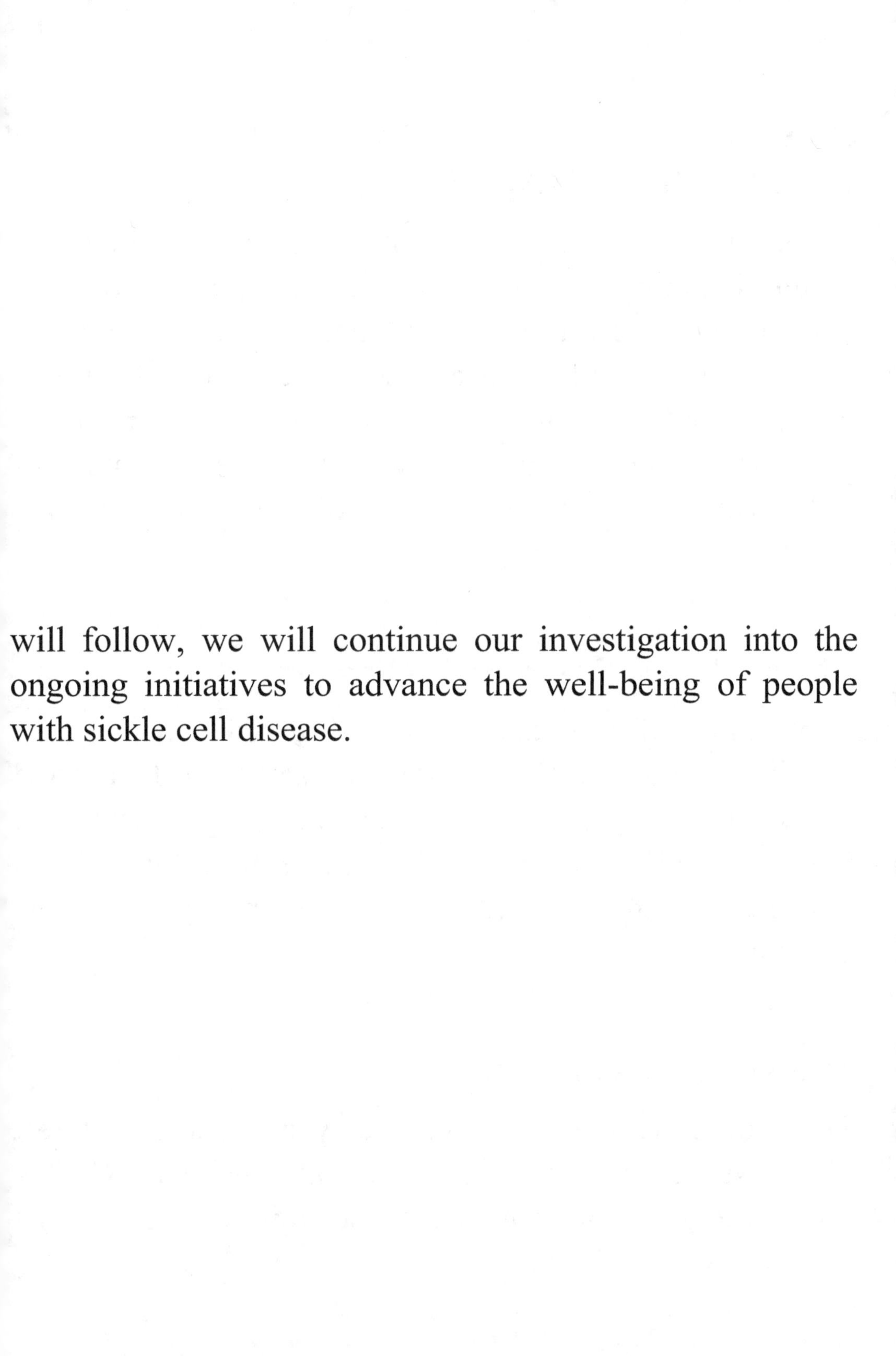

will follow, we will continue our investigation into the ongoing initiatives to advance the well-being of people with sickle cell disease.

CHAPTER 8: CLINICAL TRIALS AND RESEARCH ADVANCES

A constantly changing environment of clinical trials and ground-breaking research has been spurred by the unrelenting hunt for better treatments and, ultimately, a cure for sickle cell disease. The critical role of clinical trials, current scientific developments, and the collaborative efforts that continue to shape the future of sickle cell disease treatment will all be covered in this chapter.

Clinical Trials: Progression's Engines

The engines of progress in the field of sickle cell disease are clinical studies. These studies look at the efficacy and safety of novel interventions, therapies, and treatments. Clinical study subjects and volunteers provide vital information that directs the development of new treatments.

Trials of Gene Therapy:

Trials of gene therapy have received a lot of interest lately. Numerous gene-editing methods, such as CRISPR-Cas9, are being investigated by scientists to correct the genetic defect that causes sickle cell disease. Clinical trials in their early stages have been promising, offering hope for future treatments.

Advances in Stem Cell Transplantation:

Some sickle cell disease patients are still able to have a stem cell transplant as a curative procedure. The goals of this research are to increase the effectiveness and safety of transplantation, increase the pool of suitable donors, and lessen surgical risks.

Drugs and Targeted Therapies:

Targeted therapy and drug development also depend heavily on clinical studies. These trials evaluate how well patients' issues are reduced and their quality of life is improved by drugs like voxelotor (Oxbryta) and crizanlizumab (Adakveo).

Innovations in Pain Management:

Innovations in the treatment of pain are a hot topic for research. Given the opioid crisis, finding non-opioid alternatives to relieve pain should be a top goal. Alternative approaches, such as nerve blocks and nonpharmacological therapy, are being studied by researchers to better control pain crises.

Diagnostics developments:

Our understanding of sickle cell disease is expanding as a result of advancements in diagnostic tools and procedures. Genetic screening, blood tests, and imaging advancements can detect problems early and enable prompt therapy.

Working together and advocating:

Collaboration between researchers, medical experts, patient advocacy organizations, and pharmaceutical companies is essential to advancing research endeavors. These connections support the creation of clinic studies, data exchange, and knowledge transfer.

Global Initiatives:

Research on sickle cell disease is being conducted all around the world because it is a worldwide health issue. To address the effects of the disease globally, especially in nations with high prevalence, researchers are collaborating.

Promising Findings

Recent scientific developments have shed insight into the complex molecular mechanisms behind sickle cell disease. These revelations present fresh areas for intervention and have the power to alter therapeutic approaches.

The Way Forward

Despite significant advancements, obstacles still stand in the way of effective treatments and a cure for sickle cell disease. It is necessary to address problems including lack of access to cutting-edge therapeutics, healthcare disparities, and exorbitant treatment costs.

Cooperation, innovation, and the commitment of researchers and participants alike continue to fuel the search for better treatments and, ultimately, a world where sickle cell disease is a manageable condition rather than a life-limiting one as we navigate the landscape of clinical trials and research breakthroughs. The chapters that follow will delve deeper into the burgeoning field of sickle cell disease research and the hope it offers to those affected by the condition as well as their families.

CHAPTER 9: TREATMENT CHALLENGES FOR SICKLE CELL DISEASE

It is important to recognize and comprehend the ongoing challenges that patients, healthcare professionals, and researchers face in the fight against this complex illness as we examine the path of advancements in sickle cell disease treatment. We will examine the several issues that continue to have an impact on the landscape of treating sickle cell disease in this chapter.

Access to specialized care is restricted

Particularly in underprivileged and marginalized groups, access to specialized care for sickle cell disease continues to be a significant barrier. There are disparities in care because many people lack access to hematologists or comprehensive sickle cell disease clinics.

Medical Inequalities

The diagnosis and treatment of sickle cell disease continue to be plagued by healthcare disparities. Inequalities in health outcomes are caused by the disease's disproportionately high impact on racial and ethnic minorities and their frequent struggles to access proper care.

Lack of Knowledge and Stigma

The general public frequently has misconceptions about sickle cell disease. This lack of knowledge can result in stigma, false information, and prejudice against those who are dealing with the condition, which makes their struggles even more difficult.

Management of Chronic Pain

Sickle cell disease is characterized by pain crises, and treating chronic pain successfully can be difficult and ongoing. The opioid crisis has brought attention to issues with the prescription of opioids for pain relief and the demand for more effective pain management strategies.

Costs of Treatment and Insurance Coverage

The cost of sickle cell disease treatment, which includes prescription drugs, routine check-ups, and emergency care, might be prohibitive. A crucial challenge is making sure everyone has access to affordable medical services and medications.

Mental and Psychosocial Health

Having a chronic illness can hurt one's mental health. People who have sickle cell disease could experience dejection, worry, and tension. Resources and aid for mental health are essential yet occasionally underappreciated.

ER Visits and Hospital Stays

Regular pain crises and complications may result in repeated trips to the hospital and the ER, disrupting daily life and adding to physical and mental stress.

Clinical Trial Access

Although clinical trials raise hopes for therapeutic advances, not all sickle cell disease patients have an equal chance to take part. Participation may be restricted by obstacles including geographic location, transportation, and awareness.

Challenges of Genetic and Heterogeneity

The development of universal remedies is hampered by the sickle cell disease's genetic heterogeneity and complexity. Adapting medications to the distinct genetic profiles of individuals is a goal, but it calls for very sophisticated approaches.

Inequities in World Health

Sickle cell disease affects people all across the world, and different countries have different approaches to care and treatment. In areas with limited resources, getting access to even basic medical treatment can be difficult.

While the path to therapeutic advances for sickle cell disease is marked by optimism and success, addressing these concerns is essential to ensuring that all people with the condition receive the treatment and support they require. The continued fight to overcome these obstacles and improve the quality of life for sickle cell disease sufferers depends on advocacy, research, and collaboration.

In the concluding chapter of this book, we will look to the future and examine the opportunities and emerging technologies that may reshape the landscape of sickle cell disease treatment for future generations.

CHAPTER 10: FUTURE PROSPECTS AND CONCLUSION

We turn to the future with hope and optimism as we come to the end of our journey through the world of sickle cell disease and the advancements in its treatment. Chapter 10 discusses the promising future that lies ahead and the possibility of significant changes to the landscape of sickle cell disease treatment.

Therapeutic Procedures

The search for curative remedies is one of the most anticipated developments. Targeting the genetic mutation that causes sickle cell disease directly is a huge potential of gene therapy and gene editing technologies, particularly CRISPR-Cas9. The concept of a one-time, permanent cure for this condition grows more and more plausible as research progresses.

Personalized Medicine

Treatment for sickle cell disease is entering the era of precision medicine. Healthcare professionals can improve patient care and results by tailoring medications to the unique genetic profiles and disease-related characteristics of each individual. Personalized treatment plans have the power to alter how diseases are managed.

Gene-adding treatments

In addition to genome editing techniques, gene addition therapies are being researched. These medications include giving patients' cells a functional copy of the healthy hemoglobin gene, potentially reducing the prevalence of sickled red blood cells and their effects.

Enhanced Access to Cutting-Edge Therapies

Access to novel medications, such as newly approved medications and gene treatments, is currently being improved. The goal of advocacy and legislative changes is to ensure that all sickle cell disease patients, regardless of geography or socioeconomic status, have access to these life-changing therapies.

Patient-Centered Care

The patient will be at the center of sickle cell disease treatment in the future. Plans for comprehensive care that address a person's physical, emotional, and psychological needs are more common. Teams of collaborative caregivers collaborate to offer patients comprehensive care, thereby enhancing their quality of life.

Knowledge and Instruction

The enhanced understanding of sickle cell disease is paving the way for more empathy and understanding. Misconceptions are being dispelled and stigma is being reduced through educational programs, lobbying efforts, and the voices of patients and their families.

Global Effects

Globally, sickle cell disease is a problem, and international partnerships are expanding research efforts and enhancing access to care in areas where the disease is more common. Global initiatives aim to improve the level of treatment globally and reduce health inequities.

Continued Study

Research on sickle cell disease is an active area that is always changing. New treatment targets, diagnostic methods, and tactics are being researched currently. Collaboration among researchers, medical experts, and advocacy organizations will lead to further developments.

In conclusion, the path to medical advancements for sickle cell disease is marked by tenacity, collaboration, and unwavering optimism. Although challenges still exist, the future is incredibly hopeful for anyone affected by this condition personally and as a family. Thanks to the work of researchers, medical professionals, and advocates from all around the world, the promise of curative medicines, precision medicine, and improved quality of life is within reach.

We must keep working to overcome challenges, increase awareness, and put sickle cell disease patients' well-being first as we anticipate a time when the condition will no longer be a life-limiting one. Together, we can transform the field of sickle cell disease treatment and guarantee a better, healthier future for everyone.

We appreciate your participation in our research, exploration, and optimistic journey.

Conclusion

The story of advancements in the treatment of sickle cell disease is one of the most captivating and inspirational stories in all of medicine. This road has been marked by devotion, teamwork, and unwavering hope from its early acknowledgment in the early 20th century to the cutting-edge treatments and innovative technology of today.

We start our investigation by being aware that sickle cell disease is a complicated condition that affects millions of people worldwide. A variety of social, emotional, and physical problems are associated with it. It is also a tale of resilience and advancement—a tribute to the perseverance of people who battle the disease and the commitment of those who work to make their lives better.

These chapters have covered the genetic underpinnings, the clinical manifestations, and the historical development of sickle cell disease. We've looked into the medications and therapies used in conventional therapy that have helped many people feel better and live better. We have entered the field of gene therapy and emerging technologies, which holds great promise for precision medicine and curative drugs.

We have also addressed lingering issues, such as healthcare disparities and limited access to specialist treatment, that continue to have an impact on the landscape of sickle cell disease therapy. These issues serve as both a reminder that there is still work to be done and a motivator for us to move forward.

As we conclude this journey, sickle cell disease treatment is about to enter a new era. Curative therapy, individualized care, and a higher quality of life are all within grasp. We have arrived at this crucial moment thanks to the tireless efforts of researchers, medical professionals, patient activists, and people who are afflicted by the disease.

However, the journey is far from over. It is a route characterized by cooperation, innovation, and civic duty. To raise awareness, reduce stigma, and ensure that people with sickle cell disease receive the treatment and support they need, it is a journey that depends on all of us.

It is a journey that exemplifies the strength of optimism—the yearning for a time when sickle cell illness is a manageable condition rather than a life-threatening one. a day in the future when people with this ailment and their families will be able to live pain- and difficulty-free lives.

We appreciate your accompanying us on this adventure, which embodies the human spirit's capacity for resiliency, exploration, and change. Together, we will keep paving the way for a better, healthier future for everyone affected by sickle cell disease.